Set Your Mind
And
The Body Will
Follow

I0440490

How to Achieve a Positive Mindset
for
Life Long Fitness

RON KNESS

No part of this book may be reproduced, stored in a retrieval system, or transmitted in any form or by any means, electronic, mechanical, photocopying, recording, scanning, or otherwise, without the prior written permission of the publisher, except for the inclusion of brief quotations in a review.

This book is for **personal use only**.

Copyright © 2016 Ron Kness

All rights reserved.

ISBN-13: 978-1536831498

ISBN-10: 1536831492

Contents

Disclaimer

This publication is for informational purposes only and is not intended as medical advice. Medical advice should always be obtained from a qualified medical professional for any health conditions or symptoms associated with them.

Every possible effort has been made in preparing and researching this material. We make no warranties with respect to the accuracy, applicability of its contents or any omissions.

See your healthcare professional before starting any diet or exercise program!

The Paradox

For many, losing weight is part of their program to get healthy and live the healthy lifestyle. But losing weight is as much of a mental challenge as it is physical.

Burn 3,500 calories more than you consume in a week, and you'll lose a pound of weight (theoretically as there can be other factors involved). That is the physical part that happens as a result of a calorie deficit. The mental part is having the mindset to stay with a program that will result in reaching your weight loss goal and is the basis of this book.

In the modern age, we have a plethora of effective workouts, exercise equipment, and skilled trainers. We have ab trainers, free weights, kettlebells, resistance bands, weight machines, treadmills, bikes, rowing and elliptical machines.

We have fitness watches, gadgets, pedometers and countless fitness apps.

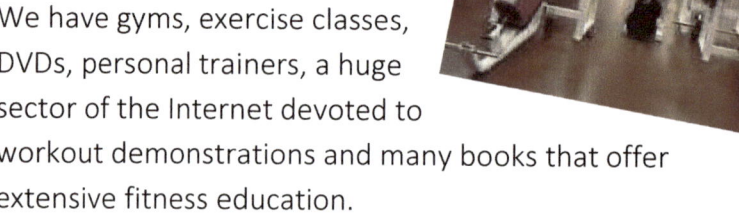

We have gyms, exercise classes, DVDs, personal trainers, a huge sector of the Internet devoted to workout demonstrations and many books that offer extensive fitness education.

But, yet, according to the Centers For Disease Control, obesity rates in the United States alone are at epidemic levels, with 1/3 (34.9% or 78.6 million) of adults being overweight or obese.

There are more people with obesity related Type 2 Diabetes than ever before.

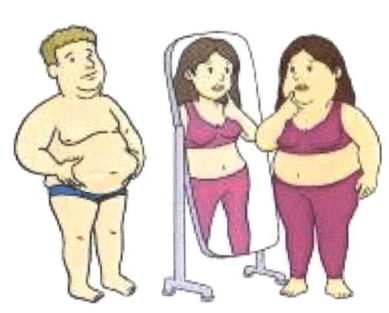

More people are dying of heart and other diseases as a result of poor lifestyle habits, such as a lack of proper nutrition and exercise than ever before.

According to the American Heart Association, 32% of adults do not engage in physical activity, which they define as light, moderate or vigorous physical activity for at least 10 minutes per day.

Why Is This So?

The simple reasons is that they don't want to!

A sensible explanation is that most people do not have the proper mindset that it takes to maintain an active lifestyle that results in fitness and good health.

Do you remember a time when you wanted something really bad and nothing stopped you until you achieved that goal?

The old saying, "where there is a will, there is a way" is very real!

Everything we do is dictated by our minds. We have incredible power to make amazing things happen, and this includes becoming fit, trim and lean individuals.

Set your mind, and the body will follow!

The Problem

The root problem for many people who spend their lives procrastinating and making excuses as to why they don't exercise is they lack the proper mindset towards it.

Typically the excuses to not workout go like this...

"I'm tired"

"I am too busy"

"It's boring"

"I can't afford a gym"

"It hurts"

Oh, and the all-time favorite "I don't have time"

But, all of these are just excuses. They really are.

The truth is that people who don't exercise don't want to. It's really that simple. They may say they do on the outside, but deep down, they do not want to change.

Another truth is that everyone can find time to exercise, and you don't need a gym to workout.

And, if we are to be honest with

Sick And Tired Yet?

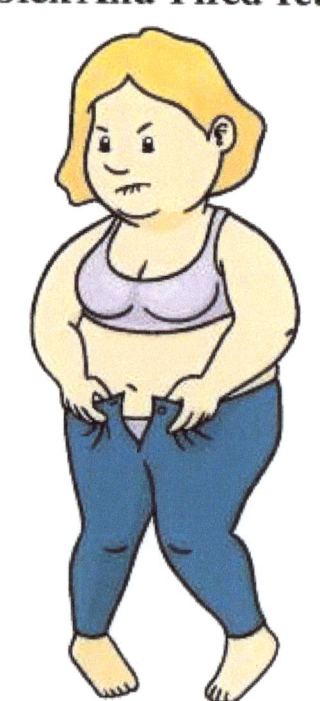

ourselves, we always find time to do the things we really want to do. Most people manage to (waste) a couple of hours sitting in front of the TV each day, but won't use some of that time to improve their health? It makes no sense to me, when you can exercise WHILE watching TV.

This is one of the reasons for the huge success of the diet industry that comes out with a new fad diet, or some new "magical" weight loss supplement every other month and people jump on it like it's a drink from the fountain of youth. It is the hope and promise of a quick and easy fix.

The reality is that achieving health, fitness and a great body takes time, effort and dedication through a sensible diet and regular exercise. There are not easy or quick fixes. It takes sweat and the desire to do it!

BUT YOU HAVE TO WANT IT. YOU HAVE TO BE MOTIVATED TO DO IT.

That Is reality.

THERE IS NO MAGIC PILL AND NO MAGIC DIETS!

But, people are attracted to the notion because it sounds fast and easy, and much easier than exercise, which they don't want to do.

In order to get fit, one must ***want to*** get fit and that begins with changing the mindset.

It is really a simple as that.

Every year people make resolutions for things they want to achieve or change in the new year. According to Statistic Brain, for the last three years in a row the #1 resolution made was to lose weight. Most of these are empty promises that will not come to fruition, because most people don't really mean them, they are just robotic statements we make because "that is what you are supposed to do at the new year."

Real behavioral changes begin with the proper mindset.

Attitude And Perception

Why is it that some people can't wait to hit the gym, the treadmill or the weight bench, while, others look for any excuse to get out of it?

Sometimes the differences can stem from different attitudes and perceptions that people have towards fitness.

Some of these perceptions are set in childhood where parents are not active and most of a child's leisure time is spent in front of the TV or playing video games – a big part of why childhood obesity rates are so high today.

Athletes have spent most of their lives, starting as young as 8 or 9 years old in training and so fitness has always been a part of their daily lives.

Some people may have had bad experiences with workouts where they experienced muscle pain the next day and it really turned them off. Understandable, but, still not a good excuse because the pain is very temporary and does go away in a couple of days.

In order to change our mindset towards fitness, we must change how we perceive it and our attitude towards it.

For any real change to take effect we must instill real habit changes that go with a new mindset that will allow regular exercise to become a part of our daily lives.

Habits

The simplest definition of habit is a thought or activity that is repeated over and over again.

The mind is, by nature, habitual. There is an inbred habit forming process in all of us that is part of our bio-wiring, and it is there in large part to help humans with one of the most important aspects of survival, which is learning.

Habits are also integral in bringing us towards something we perceive as positive or pleasurable or to take us away from something that is negative and brings pain.

Changing habits is integral to changing one's mindset and vice versa. So once you set your mind to change habits, and take actions steps to change the mindset, new habits can be formed in as little as 21 days.

Have you ever quit or started doing something and it is so solidified in your mind and your life, that the mere thought of doing it or not doing it again is an impossibility? That is a habit that has become ingrained and so behavior follows.

Athletes spend their whole lives in training, for them exercise is a regular habit and one they don't even think about, it's just a part of daily life.

Those who kick the sugar habit never touch soda. It never even occurs to them to order it, or buy it. They replace soda with other drinks and they never question it, or yearn for it because they have changed their taste so much that even one sip of that sugary drink is a huge turn off.

This is a great example of a change in habits and mindset.

Elements Of Changing Habits

Willingness And Motivation

In order to change habits you must be willing and it starts with motivation. Motivation is what drives us to do anything in life, typically there is some payoff that we wish to attain. Motivation for fitness is plentiful, you just have to be willing to go there and make the connections.

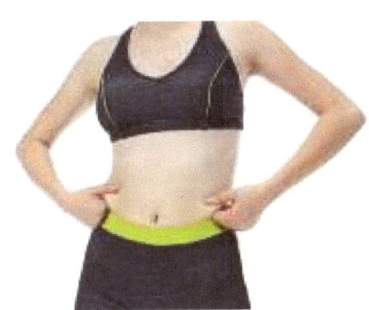

Here are some of the best reasons to get fit:

- A great body

- Better health

- To be a good role model for your kids

- Strong lean muscle tone that will ensure healthier senior years

- Wearing a bikini at the beach

- Six pack abs

- Energy and vitality

- Disease prevention

- Avoiding early death from heart attack, stroke, cancer

- Preventing Type 2 diabetes

- Preventing back pain

- Preventing arthritis in the aging years

- Strong bones to prevent osteoarthritis in women
- Confidence
- Self esteem
- Feeling of pride for achieving something great
- Feeling like a rock star when you push weight around and your own body as the sweat pours off your face
- Self-Discipline
- Wearing skinny jeans
- Eliminate joint pain
- Eliminate a variety of ailments that result from obesity
- Heart health

The connection between exercise and the payoffs listed above must be accepted if one is to make lasting habit changes. And YOU have to want to do it. Just because someone else want you to do it is not enough. The desire has to come from you. And if you want it bad enough, it will happen because you set your mind to do it.

Positive Reinforcement

One of the best ways to change habits is through positive reinforcement, so it is important to look for it and find it in fitness. Positive reinforcement is simply the reward of doing something.

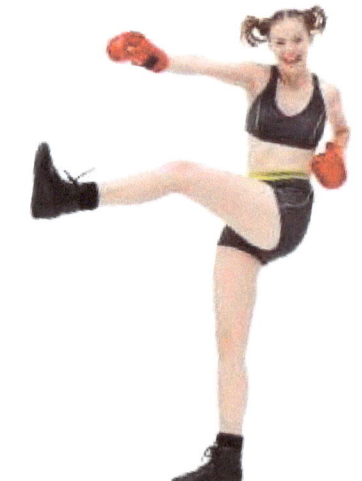

When you realize and truly accept the rewards of working out, you will want to do it.

What does positive reinforcement look like?

- Feeling some room in your jeans after two weeks of working out.
- Watching the scale numbers fall.
- Going shopping and looking for new cute outfit in a smaller size.
- Wearing clothes that you would not dare wear before.
- Feeling stronger.
- Looking better.
- Having a friend or people at the office comment on your weight loss.
- Going to the doctor and finding out that your cholesterol numbers are lower.
- Feeling lighter.

All of these and more are positive reinforcements resulting from exercises. They are the pay off. That is what drives and solidifies the changing of habits, and motivates you to keep going.

All of these help shape a new mindset!

Action Steps

Changing one's mindset and developing the habit of fitness takes action. Thinking about it can only get you so far. Action steps are necessary to reshape habits and the way we think about and perceive fitness.

And, it is also important to note that it is not a one-time event. It is something that will continue on an ongoing basis, as there will be days when you will want to give up and go back to your old ways. Remember it takes 21 days to break an old habit or establish a new one.

Identify

The most important step is to become aware of, acknowledge and accept that the reason you never exercise is because you don't want to.

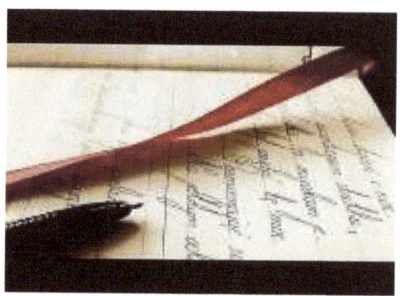

This type of conscious acknowledgement is the first step towards making change. You see if you keep thinking and believing that it really is because you don't have time, then you will never have time, and you will never allow the benefits of fitness into your life.

Identify your pitfalls in advance

- Your self-defeating thoughts and behaviors towards exercise.

- What are you strengths and weaknesses?

- What stirs you to action?

Decide how you will face them and deal with them once they come.

Commit

The second step is to make a commitment to yourself with yourself. Create a written contract. Decide that you will honor the commitment, and read that contract every single day.

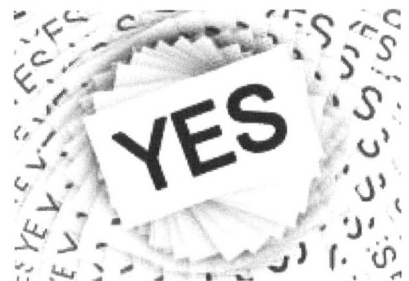

This is a tangible action step that will allow this issue to become forefront in your mind and bring it to reality. This can work wonders to stop the lies (excuses) we tell ourselves. This step also helps to plant that seed in the mind, so when we do make those excuses, we begin to see them as such.

You know yourself best, and perhaps setting personal consequences when you dishonor commitment, or perhaps it's reward, like a movie when you do, may work to keep you on track.

No More Excuses

Make a list of the excuses you typically make to not workout, and then add counteracting reality statements for each one. These should be addressed to yourself, so when you read them it will be like talking to yourself.

Keep this list handy, make copies, one for home, and one for your purse or wallet and keep it with you.

For example:

Excuse: I am too tired.

Reality: I am not really tired, it's just an excuse, besides, I will feel energized after the workout.

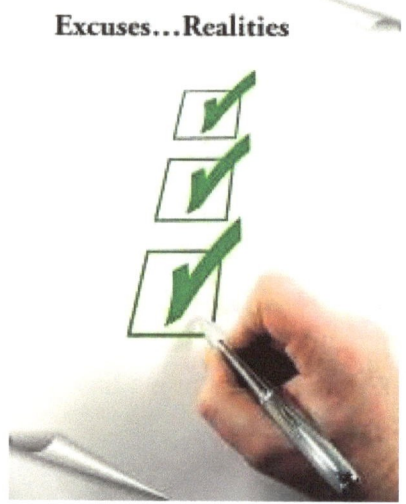

Excuses...Realities

Excuse: I don't feel like it.

Reality: Imagine how I will feel and look if I don't.

Excuse: I don't have time.

Reality: It only takes 30 minutes, much less time than it will take to watch my TV show, or to talk on the phone with a friend. I can alter my schedule, it's too important to miss. (You can even exercise while watching TV, so in reality it doesn't even take any more time).

Excuse: It's too hard.

Reality: I am a strong person, I am working hard to achieve my goals, it will get easier as I get into better shape, but if I keep skipping workouts, this excuse will always keep me from achieving the body of my dreams and sound physical health.

Continue with your own excuses and realities that make sense for you. It's also a good idea to read this every day, it will help to reprogram the mind, prevent self-sabotage and change negative thoughts and perceptions about exercise.

Positive Affirmations

Positive affirmations are sayings one repeats daily in order to achieve some type of goal. The sayings are typically spoken in present tense and can work well to re-program the mind and keep one focused on their goals.

Again, these support the changing of the mindset to stick with fitness on a regular basis.

Examples of Positive Affirmations

- I am losing weight everyday
- I have a healthy and strong body
- I love to work out, it's fun and it works
- When I work out I love myself
- When I work out I prevent disease
- When I work out I fit into my favorite clothes

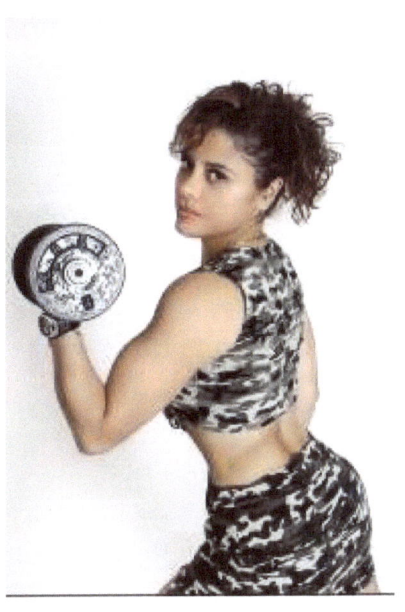

- Working out makes me feel great
- Exercise allows me to wear anything I want
- Exercise is healing
- I don't like skipping workouts
- I love how my body looks

Tangible Motivation

Tangible motivation can come in many forms. There are great motivational sayings with images online that you can look at every day to stay focused on your goals. You can print them out, look at them and repeat them every morning before you begin the day.

One of the best ideas is to print a picture of a woman or man that has the body of your dreams and pin it at home, and in the car where you will see it several times per day.

This can go a long way to remaining focused, keeping the goal you want to reach in mind and close by at all times and to keep those mindset juices flowing.

Visualization

Use the power of visualization and mental imagery. Picture yourself working out, sticking with your commitment, and following through.

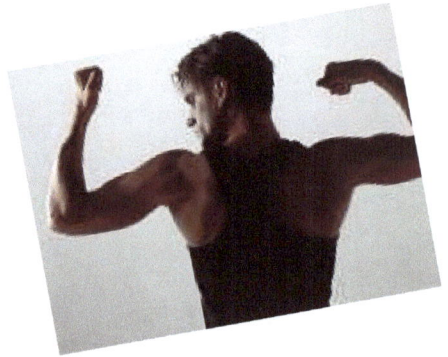

Imagine your new body.

Imagine yourself overcoming obstacles and most important imagine the feeling of pride and confidence that results from sticking with it and overcoming all the challenges.

Imagine what you can achieve and how good it will feel, and then visualize how these actions can influence other parts of your life by allowing you to realize that you can do anything you set your mind to!

The Right Crowd

Another important action step in changing the mindset for fitness is to surround yourself with fitness-conscious people. This can have an amazing influence on your perception and general attitude 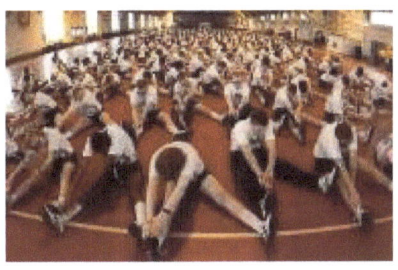 towards fitness. Those who are involved in fitness on a regular basis are true enthusiasts and they have such a positive outlook on it that it can certainly rub off on anyone they associate with.

These people are also great to workout with, because their motivation and how they push themselves can influence what you do and your general attitude towards fitness.

The opposite is also true. People with negative attitudes can make you question of you are doing the right thing. Avoid them at all costs!

Cultivate A Belief In Yourself

It is important to cultivate a belief in yourself that will drive you to overcome challenges, change habits and change the mindset.

"Yes I can" is a powerful statement. Remind yourself of it every single day. Write it on paper and stick it all over your home, one on the bathroom mirror, the fridge and anywhere else where you will see it all the time.

Celebrate And Note Success

It is important to acknowledge all successes that result from exercise, no matter how small, as they are the positive reinforcements mentioned previously that change habits and mindset!

Congratulate yourself, reward yourself, and rejoice with any of these successes:

- Lost a dress or pant size!

- Worked out consistently for a week straight!

- Lost 5 pounds!

- Increased your workout time because you feel stronger, and more fit!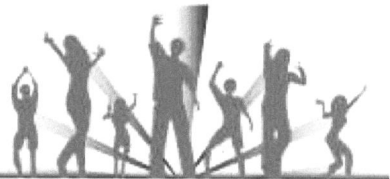

- Feeling more energy, and vitality and experiencing better sleep!

- Lost 10 pounds!

- Lowered your cholesterol!

- Had someone comment on how great you look!

- Had a family member or friend tell you they are proud of you!

- Etc...

- Etc...

- Etc...

Write them down in a journal so you can refer back to them as reminders when the excuses try to creep back in.

These are all the payoffs that blast the excuses. They are the rewards. And they are what solidifies the mindset with a different outlook on fitness.

Avoid Self Sabotage

Set Realistic Expectations

If you are new to exercising, do not sabotage your efforts before you begin by starting a workout that is beyond your current fitness level.

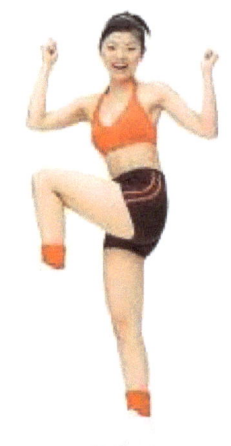

Many who begin a fitness program go all out, and choose a fitness program the in no way can sustain. They end up sore after the first workout and give it up. And if they do continue, it quickly leads to burn out that will end in quitting altogether and reinforcing those old excuses.

Take it easy and start at the appropriate level for you. Don't over reach, you will get there, just make sure you get there the right way.

Remember perception and attitude. If you start by trying to do 30 minutes of High Intensity Interval Training (HIIT) every day, you will quickly be turned off as these are vigorous workouts that you should strive for, not start with.

Realistic expectations increase the probability of success and the likelihood of obtaining them.

Get a personal trainer, they will help develop the ideal workout plan for you, one that is personable that will allow you to build up your fitness level.

Hire A Personal Trainer

Speaking of personal trainers, they can go a long way to stimulating a new mindset towards fitness. The best ones know how to motivate and encourage and can be key to proliferating the fitness mindset.

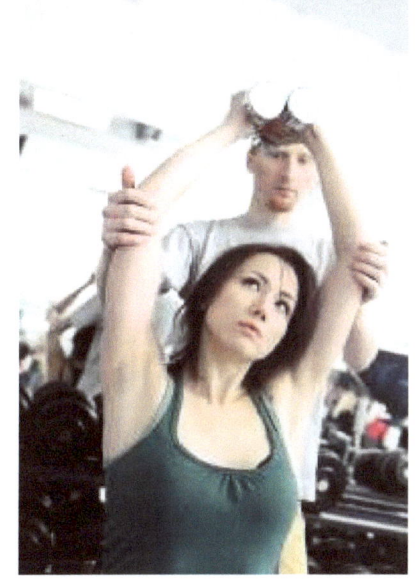

They can be incredible assets in providing that extra push that you will need to stay focused. It is also harder to make those excuses for not working out because you will have to cancel appointment and explain why you can't make it.

Find A Workout You Like

Ignore the hype of the latest and greatest and find a workout that you like. This goes back to perception and pay off that drives habit and mindset changes.

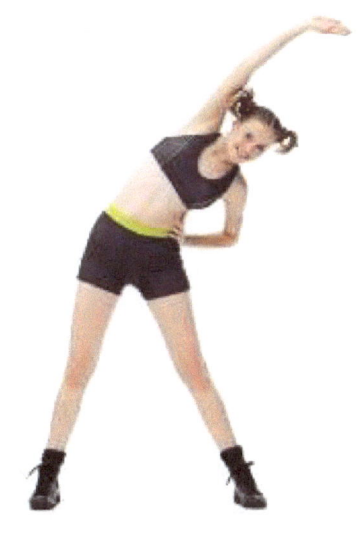

Humans need some type of gratification in order to continue a behavior. There are so many choices available today in workouts that there are no excuses or at least good ones.

Find a workout that you enjoy doing, and it's okay if you have to try 20 different ones before you land on the goldmine.

Just remember one thing, there is no "one size fits all" in fitness. And, as long as you are active and perform some type of movement daily, you are still way ahead of the majority of people sitting on the couch feeding their faces.

One Day A Time

Sometimes we are our own worst enemies. One of the best ways to sabotage your efforts is to think too far into the future, instead of staying in the moment. One of the greatest tools of success in 12-step programs are mindset slogans, like, "one day at a time" and "just for today."

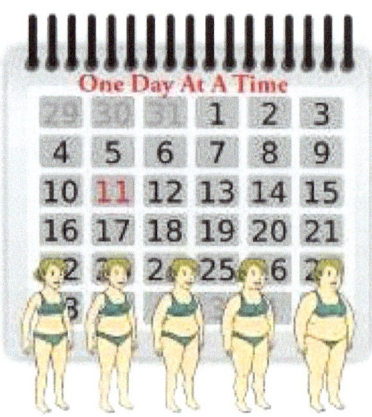

Why?

Because all we really have is today, and to think about - 30, 60 or 300 days of working out is just too overwhelming and can be a big turn off.

The only workout you have to think about is the one you will do today!

That's it.

Yesterday's is over. And tomorrow's is not here.

Is Your Mind Set Towards Your Health?

A lot can be said about the correlation between health and your mindset, while there are plenty of detractors who say different, there are plenty of studies that show it to be true.

A positive mind-set can do a lot for success in your career and in your home life, so why would the same not be true for your health?

Positive Thinking

WebMD has a wonderful article by the Mayo Clinic that goes in depth discussing the benefits of positive thinking to your health. It isn't just your mental health that improves either.

Notwithstanding the psychological benefits, positive thinking offers an increased life span, reduced risk of cardiovascular diseases, improved coping skills in times of stress, higher immunity levels, and lower rates of depression.

If you're unsure whether you are guilty of negative self-talk, just consider your inner dialogue.

- For instance, do you focus on weaknesses? Or do you consider them to be opportunities?
- Do you allow yourself to slip into a mood, or do you shake it off when you realize what is happening?
- Do you find time to exercise, or make excuses why you can't?
- Is your diet made up of healthy and nutritious foods, or do you rely on microwave meals for convenience?

- All of those thoughts can feed into a negative mindset, or a positive mindset.

If you find yourself leaning towards more negative thoughts, then just steer yourself away from them. It's an opportunity for growth.

Growth Mind Set

Health Psychology published a study, which involved two different groups being given the same milkshake, with each group being told it contained a different calorific quantity. The drink was 380 calories, but Group A believed it contained just 140 calories, and Group B that it was 620 calories.

The idea was to measure the ghrelin levels of each group after they had consumed the shakes. Ghrelin is a hormone that stimulates the brain to increase your appetite.

The group who believed their drink was 620 calories saw their ghrelin level decline sharply. Their mind set was what made that happen, not what they had consumed, as both groups consumed the same beverage.

Setting your mind towards your health and success is a sure way to truly succeed.

Plan to Succeed

Clinical Psychology Review studies have shown that optimistic people tend to be healthier on average.

Every day we are faced with decisions, consequently it is the choices we make that will ultimately affect our health. By applying positive thinking and a growth mind set, you are putting yourself in the best position to succeed, since the expectation you have set for yourself is success.

How? There are a number of strategies that you can employ to set yourself up to win.

Write it down- it might sound trivial, but keeping a journal to record your goals is an excellent way to push yourself to achieve on a daily basis. **Psychology Health** even did a study on the effects.

Whether you decide to make 3 goals every day, or leave yourself, a motivational note - do it!

Simply making a note of everything you will do in a day just so you can cross it off as you go offers such a fantastic feeling it spurs you on to accomplish even more the following day.

Be brave - if you want to do something, go out and do it; don't allow the fear of failure to prevent you from spreading your wings to succeed.

Learn - you might think you don't have time to read up on setting your mind to your health, but you probably find ways to waste your time by checking up on your social media accounts throughout the day. Instead, pick up a book that will assist you in improving yourself.

How Lifestyle Choices Determine Your Health

Lifestyle choices help you prolong your lifespan and reduce the risk of suffering from serious diseases. Making healthy lifestyle choices like eating more fresh vegetables and fruits every day or exercising at least three times a week will go a long way to improving your health.

A great example of how lifestyle choices determine your health is smoking. We are all aware of the health risks that go along with smoking, yet many people choose to smoke a pack a day. When you're smoking, the carcinogens found in cigarettes will directly have an effect on the molecules in your body. They will trigger the growth of cancer by mutating your anti-cancer genes and making them ineffective.

However, the good news is that both exercising and eating right have a positive effect on your body at a molecular level. According to an article published in *The Atlantic*, studies have shown that following a healthy diet makes the genes decrease the risk factors for heart disease. The article also mentions another study that found exercising can help transform stem cells into blood and bone cells (rather than fat cells).

Despite most people knowing about how healthy lifestyle choices can have a positive effect on their lives, they still decide to stick to their unhealthy ways. This is mostly because we are creatures of habit, and we've gotten used to eating unhealthy food and living an overly sedentary life when we were children.

Without a doubt, changing your habits can be hard, but it's something you should really consider doing to improve your health and increase your longevity. Not only will you potentially avoid suffering from some serious diseases, but you will also feel much better on a daily basis and live longer.

Many people find exercising regularly to be really difficult, but engaging in physical activity several hours a week is key to not only improving your cardiovascular health, but also improving both your emotional and psychological health.

Living healthy means avoiding foods that contain a lot of trans fats, sodium, added sugars, processed chemicals, and saturated fats, which are essentially ingredients present in the majority of the foods we constantly consume. Avoiding these foods can be quite challenging, which is why most people don't even bother trying to live a healthy life.

However, if you've never tried following a diet that provides you with all the needed nutrients, then you have no idea that all those delicious, unhealthy foods you enjoy are doing so much harm to your mind and body without you even noticing it.

Living healthy also means taking care of yourself and putting your wellbeing first. This means reducing stress, practicing relaxation, finding joy every day to keep emotional health in check and promoting brain health.

Let's ;look at some ways to convert your mindset over to a more healthy lifestyle.

40 Ways to Set Your Mind Towards a Healthier Lifestyle

1. **Get Excited:** You've finally decided to pursue a healthier lifestyle. Now it's time to get excited! Knowing that you will now begin a new chapter in your life should definitely excite you and keep you motivated. Remember from now on, you will both look and feel better ... and who doesn't want that.

2. **Assess Your Current Habits:** You cannot change habits or your mindset when making choices until you identify what needs to be changed. This is very important as it will allow you to become mindful of new and better lifestyle choices. For example, if you never exercise, start making an exercise plan. If you always eat dessert, begin to plan healthier choices, or eliminating at least two desserts a week to start, then plan on how you will eliminate more. Write down all your current unhealthy habits and then a plan of action next to each one on how you will make changes. Keep the list with you and read it over several times a day. In the words of GI JOE, "knowing is half the battle."

3. **Develop The Mindset:** In the previous step you have become aware of the problems and began to develop a plan of action for changing them, which begins to set your mind towards a healthier lifestyle. This awareness is key and you can use it to develop your mindset towards the healthy.

You will start to notice your old habits on a day-to-day basis, and you can catch yourself to choose something better. Remember the path you choose is always your choice. Which one will you go down?

4. **Get Interested In A Healthy Lifestyle:** Okay, so you've decided to start eating more fruits and veggies, and you started going for a run at least three times a week. That's great! However, repeating the same routine every week can be very tiring. Even if you really enjoy running, you can't make it the only physical activity you engage in.

    Instead, you should focus on learning as much as possible about living a healthy life. That means you should research different workout routines and try them out to identify those you like and find to be fun. Also, make sure to try different healthy recipes and spend more time cooking in order to truly appreciate the great taste of healthy food. When you enjoy leading a healthy lifestyle, it is a positive reinforcement that continues to solidify your mindset towards the healthy.

5. **Accept And Appreciate The Changes In Your Life:** As you start pursuing a healthier lifestyle, many things are going to change. Some nights, you may have to sacrifice going to the bar and having a few drinks with your friends for a workout. You'll also have to start eating less fast food and sweets. Before you even begin living healthy, it's important to realize everything you'll have to sacrifice in order to achieve your goals. This will help you deal with all the necessary changes that you'll need to make.

6. **Make Small Goals At First:** There's nothing wrong with having your first goal be losing five pounds. On the contrary, your goals should be small at first, because that will help you achieve them sooner. The sense of accomplishment that you get from achieving a goal will definitely help you stay motivated to lead a healthier lifestyle. These small changes will soon snowball into one giant change, a healthier overall lifestyle, and better choices.

7. **Be Aware Of All Of The Benefits That Come From Living Healthy:** If you find it difficult to set your mind towards a healthier lifestyle, then you should take some time to go on the Internet and research all of the healthy benefits that you can experience by living healthy.

   You probably already know that living a healthier life will help you lose weight, get you into shape, and lower the risk of certain medical conditions and diseases. However, did you know a healthy lifestyle will also boost creativity, reduce anxiety and stress, keep your eyes healthy, strengthen your bones and heart, make it easier for you to concentrate, fill you up with energy, and more? The more health benefits you know about, the more motivated you will be to stay healthy.

8. **Stop Saying 'I Should' And Say 'I Choose To':** Saying that you should start running in order to lose weight won't get you far. If you make living healthy a responsibility, then you probably won't be successful in reaching your goals. Instead, change your mindset so that you always say 'I choose to do this.'

By doing this, you will let yourself know that you're in complete control and that you're making the choice - it's called empowerment.

9. **Document Your Progress:** It doesn't matter if you lost just a quarter of a pound, you need to document it. After all, a little progress is better than no progress. Documenting how well you're doing will make you see that all the sacrifices you've made aren't for nothing, and that you are on your way to reach your goals.

10. **Surround Yourself With Like Minded People:** Nothing is more inspirational than being around people who make healthy a priority, consider this versus your friends who never exercise, drink too much and view French fries as a main staple of their diet. The gym or a fitness class is a great place to meet people that will support your efforts and help keep you in the proper mindset.

11. **Learn To Forgive Yourself:** You've vowed to stop eating chocolate, but you simply couldn't resist the temptation today. This shouldn't get you down, as it's completely understandable when it happens once in a while.

Learning to forgive yourself for a slip-up or a mistake is something you will have to do eventually, as that's the only way you'll manage to stay motivated. The only way that you will truly reverse all the effort, you put in up until this point is if your slip-up gets to you and you give up on living healthy. The slip-up was only a bump in the road, did not have any major negative effect on your overall goal.

12. **Stop Obsessing:** You definitely shouldn't stare at the mirror for hours every single day and obsess over why you aren't seeing any changes yet. If you've never been physically active or on a diet, it's going to take some time for you to see major changes in your appearance.

13. **Stop Being Embarrassed:** So what if you're overweight and everyone else in the gym is super fit. There is absolutely no reason to be embarrassed about your appearance or physical abilities. Remember, the fit people around you were also out of shape once and had to work hard to look good. They will admire you for taking action to try and improve your looks and health.

14. **Be Proud Of Yourself:** Instead of being embarrassed, you should be proud of yourself for finding the motivation to start living healthier. Know that living healthy definitely isn't easy, and most people can't do it.

15. **Make Exercising Fun:** Not everyone enjoys lifting weights or doing CrossFit; and if you don't enjoy any of these activities as well, then you simply shouldn't do them. There are plenty workout routines, and there is surely at least one that is perfect for you. The only way you'll be motivated to exercise is if what you're doing is fun.

However, if you're having a hard time finding a workout routine that suits you, you should consider starting to work out with a close friend or a relative. Having somebody by your side when you're engaging in a challenging activity will definitely make it fun.

16. **Learn To Enjoy Cooking:** Start learning which foods go well with each other. When you're bored, browse the Internet for delicious recipes. Research how to tell if the food you're buying is fresh or not. Learning to enjoy preparing a meal will make you look forward to following a healthy diet.

17. **Start Planning Ahead:** For example, start making your own healthy snacks, and always have one with you when you go to work. That way, if you ever get hungry, you'll have a healthy snack to fall back on instead of going to the vending machine and getting something unhealthy. Being prepared for every situation will make it easier for you to live healthier.

18. **Have A Positive Outlook On Life:** Being in a negative mental state will cause you to make unhealthy decisions. Many people turn to alcohol and/or junk food when they feel sad or frustrated. Know that your mental state has the power to trigger any of your previous unhealthy habits. This means that having a positive outlook on life will help you stay on the right path. When something stressful happens to you, try not focusing too much on it.

19. **Learn To Relax:** Do whatever you can to relax as much as possible. When you're relaxed, it will be easier for you to exercise and eat healthy on any given day. Excellent ways to relax include getting enough sleep, meditating, as well as eating certain foods known for giving you a mood boost.

20. **Love Yourself:** When most people who've neither followed a diet nor exercised a day in their lives decide to start living healthier, they do so because they are not happy with who they are.

No matter how you look or what type of unhealthy habits you have, you should definitely love yourself more. As soon as you start practicing self-love, it will be much easier for you to start enjoying working out and eating healthy.

21. **Choose To Eat Bright Colored Foods:** Science says that bright-colored vegetables and fruits are high in antioxidants. Antioxidants are substances that help stop or prevent cell damage caused by free radicals. Just think about the beautiful bright colored foods such as tomatoes, oranges, avocados, blackberries, and mangos. Just the thought of these foods should leave you craving for them.

    As soon as you get into the mindset in which healthy foods start looking really beautiful to you, it will become easier for you to eat healthier, further solidifying a new positive outlook towards a new lifestyle.

22. **Learn To Say No:** You shouldn't eat a pizza just because someone offered you a slice. If you're not hungry and feel like sticking to the diet that you planned, you should refuse whatever unhealthy foods someone offers you. Being out with your friends is not a good enough reason to eat something that's unhealthy. Learning to say no will prevent many future setbacks.

23. **Spend More Time Outside And Learn To Appreciate Nature:** Nothing will help you clear your head like going out for a walk in the park, especially if your job involves you sitting at a desk for eight hours. Make it a must for you to go out for a walk at least once a week ... three or four times per week is better, but once a week is a good place to start.

It will help you get prepared for all the challenges that go along with living healthier.

24. **Enjoy Your Meals:** Just because you've prepared something healthy doesn't mean that you should wolf down the whole meal while watching TV. Instead, turn off your computer and TV, and appreciate the meal your about to eat. Go with small bites, and chew for a while to really experience every ingredient. Eating like this will make you look forward to living healthy.

25. **Having A Cheat Day Is Okay:** Saying you won't eat cake during the next year is essentially setting yourself up for failure. If you're properly motivated, you might just manage to do it. However, you'll most likely fail - and that's completely okay!

   Just because you decided to start living healthier doesn't mean that you should completely forget about the unhealthy stuff. In fact, it's important (for the sake of your mental health) to have a cheat day every once in a while. During a cheat day, you can eat virtually anything you please, as long as it's in moderate portions. By having a cheat day, you will relieve yourself of a lot of stress and make it easier for yourself to continue with your diet.

26. **Take A Few Days To Rest Every Once In A While:** Just like it's hard not to eat cake for 365 days straight, it's also hard to exercise every day of the year. You probably already know that one rest day per week is totally fine (and recommended), but you should also know that taking a few days to rest periodically is totally okay as well.

This will give your body time to heal and it will make you more prepared for the following workout sessions.

27. **Try To Change The Mindsets Of People Close To You:** If you have friends who constantly eat fast food and drink alcohol, then you are probably surrounded by stories that involve these two things. Being around people like this will make it harder for you to achieve your health goals. That's why it's not such a bad idea to either try to change the mindsets of people who are close to you or drop them from being your friends. If you decide to drop them, tell them why. They might just decide to join your healthy lifestyle quest instead of losing you for a friend.

28. As soon as you get them interested in living a healthy life, you will have more motivation to reach your own goals. Simply knowing you can talk to someone close to you about the challenges of trying to live a healthy life will help you a lot.

29. **Kids Are Your Motivation:** Think about your children's health and their future, when you learn to set your mind towards health, this will teach them the same, no better motivator to start today.

When you look at some parents who are overweight and out of shape and you see their kids are the same way, you have to ask yourself if it is their environment or hereditary. In most cases, they are products of their environment of unhealthy food and lack of exercise based on their parents as role models, albeit not very good ones either.

30. **Play Team Sports:** Playing team sports is a great way to socialize while working out. Whether you enjoy basketball, baseball, or football, playing team sports is always a great idea, as they are always incredibly fun.

31. **Pay More Attention To What Your Drink:** Many people drink at least one soda and a coffee with a lot of sugar every single day. However, these drinks don't actually promote a healthy lifestyle. If you want to live healthier, the first thing that you'll need to do is make water your default drink. No matter where you go, you should carry around a bottle of water with you.

    In case you really want to drink something other than water once a day, you can go with a cup of unsweetened tea or coffee, just try to cut out (or at least down) on the amount of sugar you are consuming.

32. **Explore Different Ethnic Foods:** Don't think about healthy eating as something unpleasant. Think of it as an adventure filled with new foods and meals to explore. Make sure to try different healthy ethnic foods every once in a while. You can try dishes from Thailand, Japan, India, the Mediterranean, and any other country or area you prefer. This type of positive reinforcement continues to solidify the mindset towards the healthy.

33. **Stop Smoking:** You've started both eating healthy and working out regularly, but you're still smoking? Well, it's time to stop.

Smoking increases the risk of numerous health problems including kidney cancer, heart attack, lung cancer, and more. If you don't smoke, but are constantly surrounded by people who do, just remember that breathing in second-hand smoke is just as harmful.

34. **Stop Drinking Alcohol:** It's okay to have a drink or two at a celebration every once in a while, but if you're in the habit of drinking regularly, now would be a good time to stop. According to the ***Alcohol Research & Health*** journal, drinking alcohol regularly will have a lot of damaging effects on your brain (http://pubs.niaaa.nih.gov/publications/aa63/aa63.htm). On top of that, alcohol will also do harm to your lungs, liver, and other major organs.

35. **Stop Eating As Soon As You Feel Full:** Some people eat until their plate is empty even though they felt full halfway through the meal. If you're one of these people, then you need to learn how to stop eating when you feel full. In fact, it's even better to stop eating when you're about 90% full in order to prevent your digestive system from going into overdrive. This may be hard to accomplish at first, since most of us rely on external cues to see if we're full or not, but you should definitely keep practicing mindful eating, as that's a big part of living healthy. One way to trick your mind is to use a smaller plate. Your mind sees it as a full plate , but it ends up being a lot less food.

36. **Eat Smaller Meals:** Instead of eating two-three big meals a day, try eating several small meals. This will help you distribute energy through your body evenly during the whole day. Eating smaller meals is a healthy habit that will make you more prepared for exercising and will boost your mood.

37. **Learn To Take Deep Breaths:** Most people breathe to only a third of their lung capacity. However, considering that oxygen is a vital source of life, it's best that you learn how to breathe properly. In fact, professional athletes are all taught different breathing techniques in order to maximize their performance.

    Deep breaths can also help you relax in stressful situations. When you decide to go for a walk, make sure to breathe deeply in order to clear your mind and get the most amount of oxygen in and carbon dioxide out.

38. **Avoid Trigger Foods:** Trigger foods are essentially unhealthy foods that you always go crazy for. For some people, a trigger food is chocolate, for others it's potato chips. The first thing you need to do is identify what your trigger foods are. After you've done that, it's time to get them out of your sight. Just being around them can sabotage your goals of living a healthier life.

39. **Get Enough Sleep:** If you don't sleep enough, you will most likely compensate by eating more, and chances are that you'll overeat on junk food. On the other hand, when you get enough sleep, you won't have to snack in order to stay awake.

40. **Stop Saying That You're Too Busy:** You really shouldn't use this excuse. There are certain workout routines that literally take up only seven minutes, which is an amount of time anyone can take out of their day. In addition, if you really are too busy to cook healthy, there are plenty of restaurants that prepare healthy food.

Finally, celebrate each and every success: This is critical! Lost a pound, say hooray! Lost 5 pounds, get yourself a reward, but not one of unhealthy food. Celebrate in a non-food way.

Lowered your cholesterol, great, go out to a movie! Managed to choose to eat healthy for a week straight, say WOW, you're a rock star!

Each success is yet another positive reinforcement that continues to solidify your mindset towards the healthy.

Bottom Line

You can do this!

A great body, and good health is all in your hands. Unlike many other things in life, you have full control. **Thankfully, there are many ways to set your mind towards a healthier lifestyle.**

- **Deliberate**
- **Intentional**
- **Mindful...**

Design Your Life!

Change your mindset and your body will follow!

About the Author

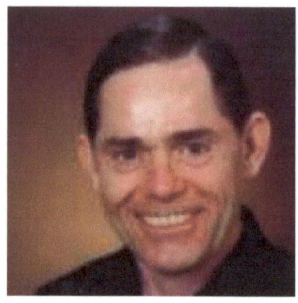

I grew up in Central Minnesota, where my parents owned and operated a fishing resort. Once out of high school I tried a couple of semesters of college, only to quit halfway through the Spring term; I decided at that time that college wasn't for me.

Then I decided to follow my father's previous occupation as an auto mechanic. I graduated from a two-year of vocational training course and worked as a mechanic. While in vocational training, I decided to join the National Guard where I eventually ended up working full-time for 32 years.

So how does all of this relate to writing? In one of my leadership schools, the instructor, who was an English teacher at a juvenile detention center, presented writing to me in a whole new way - a way that started to develop my interest in working with words.

Fast forward about 40 years and I now have over 50 books listed on Amazon for Kindle and CreateSpace.

Besides my own writing, I also ghostwrite ebooks, reports, articles, blogs and do Kindle conversions for my clients on a variety of topics.

Today my wife and I live in Gold Canyon, AZ, where you'll find me happily sitting in my office typing away on my laptop as I work on my next book or ghostwriting project . . . that is if we are not traveling on a cruise ship - our new-found mode of travel.

www.ingramcontent.com/pod-product-compliance
Lightning Source LLC
Chambersburg PA
CBHW050838290526
45792CB00001B/443